HARMONIC TWANG

HARMONIC TWANG

A DETERMINED POETS STAIRWELL TO FAITH

Logical Poetist

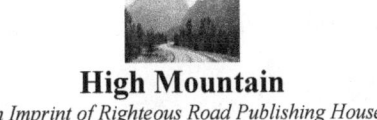

High Mountain
An Imprint of Righteous Road Publishing House

HARMONIC TWANG A Determined Poets Stairwell to Faith. First edition, November 2011

© Copyright 2011 written by Logical Poetist.

Front/Back Cover Photo: Logical Poetist, All rights reserved

Righteous Road Web Site: http://www.righteousroad.com

Righteous Road™, ™, and High Mountain™ are trademarks of Righteous Road Enterprises Inc.

All rights reserved

No part of this book may be used or reproduced in any manner whatsoever without written permission from the Author, except in the case of brief quotations embodied in critical articles and reviews.

Harmonic Twang- Printed in the United States of America.

ISBN 978-0-9831615-2-3

HARMONIC TWANG IS DEDICATED TO

Elizabeth Palmer (Great grandmother)
1901 to 1999
Virginia Robinson (Grandmother)
Virginia McCalop Mother
and last but not least
Johnnie Mae Milligan (My Aunt Teany).

These women by powerful example,
Demonstrated individually as well as collectively,
Prayer and faith would take me as far as I want to go.

They taught me about love, loyalty and sacrifice.

It is my prayer that these poetic expressions say to the world that imperfections do not impair nor provide excuses to quit. Rather they challenge one to execute the same faith my own for mothers taught me.

"Let me broaden this dedication"

To the youth in my family and worldwide

I share with you that every word born unto my soul derived from the pain of life's challenges. At times, despite praying, I felt that the universe had it out for me. There are times when you may seek refuge from life's pain yet, feel there is none.

I encourage you to pray harder and believe without wavering in whatever you are praying for. The proof that one believes is exemplified by your faith journey despite how impossible it may look.

Remember, God is always on time.
Now, that I have written my first book, it is evident that the things, I've gone through, were making valuable investments in my ability to be the literary voice of those, whose pain have silenced them forever.

Acknowledgements

To my daughter **Virginia Janai D'Raughn**, you have been my inspiration since the day you were born. Because of you, I have always found the determination to be better and greater. The guidance that you have always sought from me and your taking my advice when given, has always provided me with the power to anchor myself firmly in this world. I would not be me without you to love. Thank you "*Punkin.*"

I Love you!

I wish to say thank you to the host of family and friends who encouraged me along the way to compile and publish my words. Your expressions of the impact my literary work placed upon your spirits, is why I've followed through. Thank you all for believing in me.

Special Thanks to **Mark Thacker, Sharon Williams, Kristie L. King, Kenneth Woel** and **Michael L. Jefferson** for always being there to support, listen and provide project management.

The Art of Making Love	13
Black Woman	15
Blue Wax	18
Borrowed Sense	21
Calm	23
Change of Life	25
Daughter of the Son	27
Departing Lullaby	31
Dirty Rain	33
Do I	36
Follow	41
Grand Finale	43
Harmonic Twang	45
He Did Not Complain	46
Hint of Time	49
How Do You Know	51

In the Wind	53
Jocund	55
Light Love Life	57
Mama's Paycheck	60
Melancholy	63
Too Naked for Delight	64
Nanas and Grandmas Gone	66
Necessary Beats	71
Seasons of Change	74
Self's Song	76
Soaking in Somber	78
Soul	79
Sour Apples	82
Splinter	84
Sweet Molasses	85
Unsolved	87
Wages of Truth	90
Waiting	92
White Collar Worker	97
Window of Anticipation	99
Insensitively Intense	101
Spirit's Quest	103

The Art of Making Love

Peel back the blanket of her disguise
See truth behind what she denies
Never see her truths as lies
Kiss tears from each corner of her eyes
Don't be the reason she ever cries.

Caress the softness of her skin
Compliment the good she holds within
Listen when you want to speak
While she is talking, stroke her cheek.

Reference back to her what she has told
Watch as her trust simply unfolds
Stare deep and glaringly into her eyes
They are the windows to her soul.

What you see is what you get
Never walk out or become upset
For every part of her you discover
Seek understanding, don't run for cover.

Take time to hug, hold and caress
Although she excites you
Give here affection instead of sex
A woman wants to be appreciated
For her physical body yes,
Most importantly, her intellect.

Get into her mind
Study her library of thoughts
File them alphabetically
Within your heart
Recollect often
what you've been taught

Express passion and desire
Seek her internal place of higher
Place your lady at the top of your list
Always give your tenderness

When lying down with her day or night
You'll find it to be the ultimate flight
Love never starts between the sheets
And is great when laced with proper sweets

If your intimacy seems to be a wreck
It's likely you've just been having sex

Black Woman

The Black woman
Could never be confined
By mere words
Webster does her no justice
She is a soul of indescribable power

Black woman, do your thing

You are sensitive and strong
Yet have become successful
In the midst of your failures
You bathe in the sun of your family
They are the radiance of the sun in you

Black woman, do your thing

You work and never tire
Setting aflame stereotypical beliefs
indicating you are the weakest link

Black woman, you are who starts
and finishes the chain

Black woman do your thing

I noticed your hands black woman
as you dropped to your knees.
They were folded. Utterance of prayers,
Blessings of mercy came

P
O
U
R
I
N
G
down upon your children

As a result
Black woman
You induce power

Black woman
Who else besides you
Peels the skin off the truth
and gets everyone together?

The weather is dependant
Upon your forecast

Black woman
You spew the tone
of leadership with your
dignified confidence

The world cannot make sense
of your Poise attitude
How you say so much
Without ever saying anything
There is none more worthy

No more of a misinterpreted being
Than you beautiful
Sister and Queen
Than Mama
Than Nana
Or
Grandma
Who is gone
Than me

Black women
We will always do our thing
Don't hate us, love us
Accept us

We are the ones praying
Holding up spiritual walls
Preventing those falls
down into bottomless pits

Our prayers release an epiphany
So, just stand on the sidelines
clapping and shouting...

Go on Black woman
Do your thing

Blue Wax

She sat at her marbleized table
Pondering her life
Years seemed to wipe away some war stories
Others manufactured poetry and plays.

Her writing over the days
gave new definition to her pain.
Before causing her back to cave.

Yet, as she sat on this day
feeling a nagging resurface of history
that seemed to be blistering her soul
It burned like fiery coals
and took hours to form ash
So, she lashed out with a scream-

She lit a candle and watched the flame dance
Its rhythm seemed to be singing her blues
So, her tears began to fall
Each one hitting the flame,
Refusing to aim
any place else other than its reality
The reality that the pain
Never, really disappears.

Recycling of camouflaged aches
reminding her still they're alive

Lying dormant in her safe place
That's her literary expressions
Of poetry or plays.
What happens if
She experiences writers block
As an actor, stage fright?
She simply fears
She appears naked to the entire world
As Eve was when she ate forbidden fruit
Recognizing along with Adam
She too, was without clothes

Her tears flowing... knowing
if writers block stays too long
She too, curses the world
She too, disappoints her Creator
Just like Eve.

So she forces herself to scribe
As she glances forth and back
Eyes piercing the burning candle
Her tears, still falling into the flames

Sizzling... As she watches its rhythm
She realizes surely, she's not to blame
Her epiphany birthed upon pages
She is comforted by her pen
the candle releasing a scent
Very calming in that clarity came
Pain is met to be remembered
For it teaches, reminds, and strengthens.

Although, by pain resurfacing at times
Feels inconsiderate of time,
Is uncomfortable
It is evident that now she stands.

She is 5'3 and the world views her small
Yet the universe deems her tall
The universe knows that she rules
The universe, in its sole existence
Defined why she had to "go through."

She is forever great and
made even greater
Each time the moon turns
Her Stars churn like butter
She is smooth, she is rich
She is pure
Despite all uninvited
Violations
As life is Karma
Parallel the universe
She... is Mother.

Borrowed Sense

Buried deep inside the heart of love
Often, is a feeling of fear
A passion for something or someone
Control becomes impossible to steer

Undelivered yet, received
maintaining its own receipts
Instructions, not included
Inside the box
Love, not just casually passing by

Instead rushing straight to ones heart
Equation containing
2 powerful souls
Two beautiful spirits,
Totaling, one force of love
Birthing a vision
In to fruition
Includes the powerful two

Unsure of the appropriate action;
Should the powerful two divide
Knowing deep in their heart
Wishing "power two" multiplies
Wisdom and Grace
If sought they'll surely find
Love tales of yesterday
And love tales of today
Just a difference sublime

Mates successful in preceding times
Tell tales of how they've collected their years
Freely sharing loves experience.

Intelligence and Wisdom is listening
True Love means working
Compromising and accepting

Relationships are very intense
People can change
True love will exercise patience
And it does pay to borrow sense.

Calm

Time just passing
It's only what's lasted
to confirm
One's soul has grown
Hopefully wisdom
Can remember
the long way home

Never free of memory
It shall, but remain
Seek life not through
Another's eyes
Nor thoughts through
another's brain

Realize ones fears
Release ones tears
Be certain of existence no more
Gently proceed forward
Dance on this planets floor
Dance the last dance
Kiss the last kiss
As if it's the first
day of love

Never regret anything
When you've continued
to look above
Definitely never regret
A title such as LOVE

Coldness produces
Wholeness, within a storm
Razor-sharp, whirling winds
Spins the air it breathes

Panting, gasping, panting
Indicates it's time to rest

Storm now at a settling calm
Winds surrender its
biting edge
Once rough as an un-pruned hedge

Light burning forevermore
Flames of everlasting fire

Faint sounds of crackling sand
While napping by the
Sea's calm shore
Giving birth to new desire

Change of Life

One hundred six degrees rules
Hot sun screams
Ceiling fan cools
Jazz playing
hips swaying
Feeling just right
If only the mood remains steady
Prayer for a harmonious night
Flame burns
wax drips
Pauses in mid air
Mint tea
Tingly lips
Steel Daggered stare
Brown eyes bleeding
Hazel tears
Multiple colors
Blatant display of change
Present metamorphosis
Internally re-arranged
Completely changed her
Imposes a larceny
Of time

Untimely
dictation
of her world
She is left
To ponder why

Does the universe
Still, hold her securely
in its arms
Are her powers as strong as
Wonder-woman
Is she still delicate like a butterfly?
She turns to the mirror, takes a deep breath
And says...
I AM simply the next level I-

Daughter of the Son

Stopped in to check in
Have not written
Let's see, it's been
A while my friend
Here on this space,
in this place

-It May be true,
did however pay dues
to the journal.
My favorite place
to safely state
what I feel on most days.

My sun's rays
Blazing poetic sages
setting them into flames
As I-
want to remain free
Don't care to be seen
in my vulnerability
No rusty rain to drop on me.
Speech not always about freedom
Sometimes it just wants to be
E X P R E S S E D
Particularly if one just wants to address
Who cares about being on time
Lots on my mind

After all I am a
"Logical poetess"
Posing in my bliss
And if you've missed
Any of what I'm saying
Truly you are not paying
attention to the realism within
We all feel this way sometimes,
not that we're trying to hide
Anything
Just wanting
to be heard,
Not, necessarily seen.

We call it our privacy;
Only those, privy
Depths of spirituality
can enter, on these days
During these lit nights
Upon this phase
When my sun's rays
Set afire
That desire to just be alone

There was NOTHING cold about me
Then
Which is really now
In my endowment
As a writer
It all started when I was forced to be a fighter
In my youth-

Truth is
Writing is my empowerment;
Certain folks tried to destroy my innocence,
Rob me of a destiny
GOD has planned for me.

No, worry
Could not stop me
Not only,
Did GOD... design me
He is in control
Of my destiny
Therefore I was made stronger,
And better,
Folks stood in awe of
My phase's finale
Prior being completed
There were plots of serious destruction
Disruption and infraction became of what they feared
I'd ultimately become
Powerful sum infrangibly
Prevailed

Still my total self was formed
and there is no denying
GOD said, "No, my daughter!
You are as always intended to be
SUPREME BEING
I shall deal with them
They shall see you

I will prepare a place for you
In the face of your enemies
They will understand...

My command
That you walk toward them
With love
They will bow
In sorrow and shame
for what they have done.

Know my daughter
Although, you have suffered
Combat
Your battle is already won.
Your sun's rays
Blaze poetic sages
Setting lost souls aflame.
Those who follow once you are long gone
Shall not, just hear your name but know
Also
YOU are
Daughter of the SON of MAN.
Final documents shall read,
"Failed attempts"
YOU rose still as
Daughter of
The SON OF MAN
Just as I,
GOD had planned!

Departing Lullaby

Backdoor of goodbye's
Grand baby cries
Mimi, too has tears
In her eyes.

Genuine love
Sustain our hearts
Seal the trust that
we must we will
meet again and again.
My
First and only born child
One boy, one girl you returned
Two, precious gifts back me.
Magical multiplication;
You times Two.
My grandchildren
Girl– summer
Boy– fall
PLEASE...
Promise mama you'll
kiss them often and
mention my name
between calls.
I love you ALL

Thanks for the memories;
Sharing of your
Beautiful smiles,
Chimes to my heart
Sing a lullaby as we depart
For now and until-
We meet again.

Dirty Rain

Wear a mask
rubber smile
upon an iron face.

Sew a dress
of beautiful silk
spoiled with
Un-removable stains

Sipping from a glass
Half-full
filled with dirty rain.

Tore a heart, piece by piece
Injecting it with pain.
3,000 miles
for the sake
of love?

Placing shattered pieces
In to an empty cup;
Shook it
Stirred it
Until, thought it to be sweet
Poured it slowly,
It's looking lumpy
tastes like sour defeat-

Continued trying
Kept denying
That this love is
Not very good.

Unsavory flavor
Praying it stews
As it should;

Appease affliction
Not accepting
Love has lost
It's way.

Two hearts,
One soul,
Can make it
If they try
Sweeten up
That dirty rain
Do not dare deny

All hasn't been given
Much has been stolen
From an, already,
desolate place.
Don't wear that mask
Or iron smile upon your
Beautiful face.
What appears done
May be reborn

Should honesty reappear
Do not blame,
Nor deny,
Pay tribute
to wonder years

If the student
Were, not ready, the
Teacher, would not
have appeared

When the lesson
has been taught
Just as quickly
as it came,
Blessings
for all those involved
Is collectively
gained

Yet may leave
the glass
Half-full
Filled, with
Dirty rain.

Do I

My question is, do I?
Do I place a smile
upon your face,
upon acting according
to style & Grace?

Do I

Do I
seduce your heart
with my gentle smile
when I say to you,
"Stay a while?"

Do I

Do I
Stimulate your intellect
with my dialogue,
steal your attention
from that catalog?

Do I

When I ask please
turn that TV down,
If I am not looking
will you frown,
Or, do I interest you in engaging me?

Do I
Entice your mentality
To, sit and simply dream with me?
Do I

Do I
massage your mind
when we converse
discussing plans to elevate
Achieve the dreams
we hold within
Brief spells of time
we spend?

Do I

Do I
Move your soul to a place
Unlike anyplace else
You've ever gone
when I take the time
to burn your favorite song?

Send it via email
when you least expect

like during a meeting
Or while you stand in line
writing a check?

Do I?

Do I
Break into your heart
With the things I write,
Just like a thief in
the middle of night

Do I
Engage your attention
As I drag my pen across
Pink lined paper
Making it safer for tears to
cleanse your soul...
Simply because you sit alone
reading something I wrote

Do I

Do I
Intercept you
like a football game
On Thanksgiving Eve,
because, what I've written
Is just that deep

Tell me, is it a touch-down
Did I score

Plenty more
I am willing and wanting to give
you. A delicious dessert

I aim to please you,
Satisfy the sweet tooth
Of your spirit

Do I
Connect to your reality when
I write about the paralysis
of this life;
how it has handicapped innocent hearts
made them afraid to feel

Do I
Enhance, or even appeal
to your wondrous thoughts?

Do I
Make you seek within your
Own soul an opportunity
to reach for more?

Do I
Encourage, inspire,
promote your desire to
make the necessary amends
to a long, lost friend

Does my writing,
daily blogging
make clear what I am trying to do;

to heal or repair your hurts and pains,
set you walking
in brand new shoes,
Un-worn, life not torn
Perhaps a newly born you
I sure hope I do.

It's the only way if you say
that when I create these poems,
these columns,
I move you to greater heights of love,
passion and determination
to make right what has been
wrong for far too long.

Accomplishing my own goals
to penetrate souls.
Gifts of spoken words;
words that make you laugh or cry,
yet healed from the outside.
I need to know I've entered you –
challenged you – to be better, do more
and make a difference.

Awaken your obligation
bring into fruition
your own purpose.

Tell me, because it inspires me
to know that I inspire you.
So humbly I ask Do I?

Follow

No need to search anymore
He has opened the door
Your journey, be sure, does entail
Forever more.

Eternity –
That's the business He's in.

It's simple
Follow him you win
Don't just bathe in sin
Seek refuge in the bosom of Him
Let him guide your steps
help you reach depths
Unforeseen
How will you hold
the pounds of gold
He has in His plans

Use your hands
to build His kingdom
Your kingdom
Will come
from your building.
Be of a serving mind
Smile and have fun
While giving remember
Keep your mind
On His ways

His ways
not your ways
His thoughts
not your thoughts
Remember
His eyes are watching
Your heart-
Use it to utter your request
Of His holiness
Stay faithful to your request
"You shall be blessed"
Rebuke all temptations
The sensations of Christ
Lack euphoria
His promises
Will provide
water
He wants to
take you higher
He is the Messiah
The Alpha and the Omega
Who else could finish
Before, they started
If you know one like Him
produce them.
I thought not –
Jesus is all that

Grand Finale

Leaky pen, torn pages,
representation of soul's sages.
Shattered emotions, dry bones,
Defines wisdom, defies ages.
Desperate voice crying aloud
Experiences... few, to be proud
Strong hands of hard work,
Smiles equal minimal pay.

Raging ,memory, wrinkled roses.

Internal butterflies,
metaphoric, vision helps hide
Alidade captures the truth inside,
Behind all the isms and false defines.

Attempted robbery, of spiritual high,
Lies... lies while denial cries.
Streaming tears from soul's flask,
embellished result.

Bask-
Leaky pen still extend,
pages whole, emotions blend.
Torn no more, healed scars,
Lubricated bones Un-sore.

Age now births to wisdom,
Soul sages, baked pages
Setting stages,
Romantic release
Teach
Knowledge increased
Meditation displayed answers
Revelation unveiled exposition
Elation sophistication

No more judgments
God says sufficient
No more racing
Gracefully pacing
Humbly giving
Mightily living

Harmonic Twang

Sweet breath warming ones neck,
Oily palms, caressing arms

Wind chimes tickle the tips of lobes
Drum symbol of beating hearts
Articulate rhythmic souls

Time... uncalculated sum
Passing presence by
Erases the equation
Destiny is now Eternity
Contest of faithful supply

Hidden treasures captured under stream
Beacon of light, solid beam
Penetrating words, silence spoken loudest
Volcanic outpour of molten rock
Soft texture somehow hardest

Crystallized glass
Shimmies of internal glare,
Awed stare, an empty chair,
Missing link a broken chain
Obscured wink
Epiphany of unintended sermonized cold
Once a Drum Symbol of beating hearts
Once articulate rhythmic souls.

He Did Not Complain

Listen to my story
This lady screamed to me.
Soon undergoing
another procedure.
Previously, I've had...
three-
Surgeries
"My friend..."
"I am scared"
She confesses to me.

Listening closely, letting her express
all she needs to free.

As she is speaking,
I am wondering,
"How do I encourage her heart?"
Reliant upon my own faith
dependent on my God.

When she finished talking
I asked, "Do you believe in him?"
Speaking very swiftly
She answers "I do"
As much as I believe in Sin
I asked, then why
Walk in "fear filled" shoes?

I pray and pray.
Frustration passionately
in her voice,
Shouting loudly she exclaims,
Still I have bad days!
This woman forgot about choice
She states she does not understand
Where God is in my life she says
Why pray when still I feel so bland?
I replied when all fails
Prayer is the one thing that still stands

I began praying a faith increase
From the epitome of my heart
Asking Lord help her to believe
I commanded her to cry out
"Only you Lord can cancel
this wretched place.
Lord Restore my life
With Mercy and grace
Pick me up from off the ground
Give my peace
Keep my spirit Safe and sound

More and more, her passion grew
Feel the prayer breaking through
Pray, my Sister, yes do pray.
DO NOT however leave out faith
It is impossible to please God without-
He's canceled fear, removed your doubt.

The only way you will feel alone
Is if you relieve Him of His throne.

Children of God we will always be
Sons and Daughters of the King.
It really is not complicated
Your heart, your soul
"Jesus The Christ"
All integrated.
Believe and confess
from thy mouth.

Jesus came
Died for you, and
He was put to shame
Bared stakes unto his
hands and feet.
He did not complain

Thank Him, praise Him
All the time
Don't dare sit and whine.
Envision your life thru spiritual sight.

Pray, pray and never stop,
Without faith One cannot Please God.

Hint of Time

To dream the impossible dream,
Be loyal to ones vision,
to understand that clocks
don't represent time
Nor dictate course of action.

Oh, but a clock can be a distraction
if you watch it moment to moment,
or an infraction on your time because
it imposes an anxiety attack upon you.

Now you're going be late as
you cannot be calm – you must now
take some time, to relax yourself.

Behaving like a timed bomb-
You know that if you show up
with your adrenaline high
you will fumble...
may tremble when you speak.

Risk giving misinformation do
to a memory freeze
Clocks actually steal your time,
have you ever thought about that?

Next time you stare at a clock,
remember the sun, moon and stars.

Keep better track of time
Definitely keep your peace

Let the sun light your way,
the moon reveals a phase
and the stars direct your path.
Dream the impossible dream
Ease forward and never look back

How Do You Know

When you love,
love so deep
How does one know
What is on another's
mind?

Enter the room,
tummy fills
with butterflies
Moment is sublime.

Feels as if
something's wrong,
Ask the intension
Access blatantly denied
Shut out from love's
Own truth
of what is buried deeply
inside.

Belief that
togetherness
and-
Forever is
what the future
holds.

Summer is winter-
Brisk and unusually bold.

Compromising
no longer works,
It appears to have
grown old.

Unsure if
It's really okay
simply to exhale.

How can one determine
day to day,
the boat is set
to definitely sail?

How does one know
from time to time
If love is silver, copper or gold
No one REALLY knows...

Go for the journey;
As you travel
You're learning,
Another's true intension

If Luck is on your side
you begin to know fact from fiction
All one can do is ask the question;
Is this love for real this time
Or just another depiction?

In the Wind

Extending my hand
and heart to you
call you my friend.

How does that happen
with such truth,
such distance
in the wind?

Time's gone by,
events happening
from every end

sharing as much
as time allows,
through the distance
of the wind.

I trust the sun
to warm you,
trust God
to keep you
safe and sound.

Believing in Him
for deliverance
of anything
that attempts
to bring you down.

Wherever we go,
whenever we meet,
if ever or never
our souls blend,
my prayer is that
you shall always know
How grateful I am
that our friendships' grown
via the distance of the wind.

Jocund

Looking forward, not behind
knuckles just keep writing
unspoken words push beyond
what internally it's fighting...

Found warmth within a smile.

Flames of ignited passion,
How powerful the reaction,
opinionated non facts,
cracks upon ones back,
no slack no unwritten acts
stand up, don't dare sit
Don't stop and never quit.

Refuse to
say the word... "Shhh..."
Ask the question

Curiosity shall pay
just may, like what
it has to say...

Going to be spoken any way

Reasons exist, chances missed
insist on a change of season
Breathe in, Ease in,
to that place where loved.

Have fun, Laugh, Live.
Make life a playground
Always rise above.

Live life. pay it forward,
And, in full
Take no shortcuts,
no corners, and
do not ride a bull
Laugh extremely loud
Now Or all the time.

Even when melancholy
Wanes in.

A life that fails to smile
Sometime
Is a life that failed to win

Light Love Life

Expose yourself
I have seen you
yet do not know
who you are
As I am telling you
many things
about my inner being
interior décor
uninformed
of what you'll use it for
live in the trust
of another's being?
fear blocking life's blessings

It is dark
and scary in this place
of fear
Somehow-
unafraid
Am I
to expose my light.
Unafraid for light
to expose my depth
Comfortable with my natural high
for when others walked in fear
JESUS wept

I will not force
tears from His eyes
Cry instead, will I
He suffered for me
At His own expense
spiked crown
upon his head
every inch of flesh
His entire body bled

No more suffering
for my sake
Cannot afford to
be afraid
Because of
His sacrifice
My way's been fully paid

An un-wavering faith
Held inside
Life not always right

At times great days
Bare some troubled nights
GOD says
trust in HIM
walk through darkness
in to light

You're not loving
if you're not protecting

Not exposing
if you're hiding
just an unknown
Soul un-abiding
not really living
if you are afraid
of just LOVING-
Disappointing...

Defeating-
Almighty Lord's true meaning
not even seeing
that in which HE is giving

Your light
your love
your life is moving
fast
no where
going

unaware
that you are defacing
GLORY
So sad;
"Bleeeeeeeeeeeep..."
End of your story
You left no legacy

Mama's Paycheck

Mother cannot truly be defined
She is the Universe
The most diversified
of all life form

She formed life

When young
we do not understand
mother's role
We view her
as a disciplinarian
at times a nurse
other times as a teacher
or librarian
She is even a preacher

Look into her soul
through her eyes
Yet
ever does she
allows us
to see her cry
She holds back the tears
as she assumes
the pain of those
she loves

Smiling
as here spirit
and body
take on every possible task

She'll never ask
for a lending hand
yet shares diligently
with both of her own

Mother knows
before we face trouble
that we will
So she is injured internally
while warning us
She is dressed in armor still
often with ease
We reject her advice
We think our way
is better
We accuse her of being
old fashioned
un-cool
Not once remembering
she has already traveled
a road less traveled by us

SHE IS NO FOOL!

Mother
How could we ever repay you
for the countless times
that you have given of yourself
without consideration
of you-
Always thinking
of Everyone else
It is impossible to describe you Mom

Your imperfections so perfect
in the eyes of your children

So to repay you
for all that you have been
and all that you have given
I took all of your advice
not a moment too late
The reward for what
you've given unto me
I stand Tall as what you made me
and that is
simply GREAT!

Thank you

I LOVE YOU

Dedicated to you – MOTHER

Melancholy

When words suspend into air
no time to seize withdrawal
For all we know we're at the end
there will be no time tomorrow
Moment in time is short for sure-

Time...
Never guaranteed
Live for the greatness
love through all challenges
Faith... commands a mustard seed

All may be lost
gone and never to be found again

Lessons won
Totality still whispers secrets (silent pause)
of an accounted blessing

Too Naked For Delight

A Black woman can not be summed up
by any created words
I know because I am one ...
Black woman

Learned to be successful
through the experience of my failures
Lived new adventures to their exhaust
Determined never to repeat those old tired mistakes
It is hard to do

Truth is there are lessons to be learned
And once you've done the same old slip
after being shown the result
that is truly a mistake indeed
Good thing about making them is that
you can always learn from your mistake

It's like raking your soul then passing it to the youth but,

It is by no means, limited to just them.
I encourage ALL folk to learn from those
that have lived longer than them

Avoid taking things personal and you will catch on;
I don't sugar coat nothing mainly,
Because I don't want young folks to get addicted to sweets,
Even soil is black and strong, without it plants cannot grow
Try sprinkling seeds into the concrete

One person challenged Black strength
Tried to make a fool out of me and what I say
I watched as they tried to mix black with white
Of course all they got was grey
I just laughed
Angrily they asked "What's funny gal?"
I replied with dignity, my head held high
That you needed "BLACK" to get that
Now ain't that too naked for delight

Nanas & Grandmas Gone

Heavy heart
Bruised inside
Pain extended out
Gentle loving words No More
Now a scream or shout

Grandma and Nana
did it differently
had their own
style and grace

Hands that bathed you
prayers that saved you
tied your kinky hair,
bundled you up and
took you place to place

Children now
Sad for them
Their Nanas, their Grandmas
are so very young
Not taking the time
to teach their babes
Not even trying to watch their tongue

These precious children
What will they do
when faced with tough choices
as we know they will –

Having not taken time
to show them life
beyond a window's sill

Nana and Grandma
made hot meals
early in the morn
ready for a belly full
Awake since crack of dawn

Prayers said
teeth brushed
So when called
to the table
children rushed
ready for hot
cooked food
Because God is able
To be sure that
there was structure
Nana and grandma
sat and ate with us too

A set of four
deep eyes; lurking
our every move
Table manners
must be obeyed
better be watching what you do

Sunday morning
no time to play
eat up, soon time
for Sunday's school
To the Church house
we must go to hear
the preacher preach
Messages always consistent
with what Nana and Grandma teach

Do unto others
what you wish them
to do unto you
Don't steal or
fill your mouth
with lies always tell the truth

Nana and Grandmas of today
Where have your courageous spirits gone
To stand firm and show loving examples
while teaching right from wrong

It's not right that you curse at the children
while expecting them to understand
What happened to
"tanning their backside"
with a gentle loving hand

Nana and grandma
just because you're young
and do not look your age

does not negate responsibility
for you to set the stage
Wish everyone
could have the Elders
that I was blessed to have
in my life
Being strong examples
of Grandmothers
while being
an awesome Wife

Pray, pray for the young
Pray, pray we must
for the Elders too
Somehow everyone
is all off course
The children
they are lost
And lacking of a clue

On the streets is where
they're seeking love
No more backyards
with swings

No more gardens
filled with tomatoes
ears of corn, sweet yams
Turnips and Collard greens

Nana and grandma
in this day and time
not focused on a mortgage
not trying to save a dime
Who, will pay for college
Where shall the children go

Nanas and grandmas
Stand up step up
and do take back your role

Grace responsibility
back into your hands
Save our children
your children
Most children
have seemingly
lost all hope-
If you don't do it
Ultimately you are the ones
leaving them to guns and dope

Necessary Beats

What great work is really done
if hurt is inflicted on even one
soul

One seeming worth
less than one penny
Least multiplied by many
has little ability
to purchase anything of value
Decreased is the quality
of life least failed
to say something powerful
through actions

See, the fact is people talk
while sitting down
yet it's walking the talk
that crowns a head
glorious

Truth is, some things don't come
quick as a matter of fact
easily gained easily sick
regurgitating sorrow rather
manifesting solid tomorrows
guaranteeing security

Saddest seen, is a
dream come true today
lost by tomorrow's eve
Now the dreamer is
left to grieve and their story goes like this...

Once upon a time
I used to have a life of abundance
Man, you should have seen my mansion
full of beautiful things

Countless rings were right here
in this mahogany jewelry box
Oh, but that was long ago

But I'll show you
I'll gain it all back again
Not realizing the real sin
was poor management

See it was that senseless dreamer
that thought that they were the manufacturer
of their own talents and destiny
Now I don't propose that
One should serve the same God as me
but, I tell you

You better sure have a sense
A higher reality than man
Especially higher than self

That kind of vanity will surely
bring you to the mirror
and no where else can you run
when face to face with that truth
I think I've made my point
but before I go
Listen to the youth
Can't count them out
shut them down

If courageous enough to hear
their voices
Your heart will beat to
Rhythmical, true future sound

Seasons of Change

Suddenly life just changes
feeling of a sudden shift
everything just re-arranges
Un-hemmed irreparable stitch
hands of the clock
representative of time -

seems to be running out
if blessed with more
be sure to dance laugh
and shout-

Life is a precious gift
time meant to be shared
yet many treat time as if
it lasts forever
Many just don't care

The sky is soft and blue
containing thousands of clouds
in all of its peacefulness
It speaks so very loud
rain falls on everyone
It's no excuse to be rude or mean

Winter promised windy days
Summer pronounces green
Now Fall, it demands change
and Spring is when change is seen

Each season of life brings purpose
a contribution not instantly understood
Time sometimes runs out
whispers "it was all for good"

Epiphany speaks in relative form
what is displayed to the heart
Was it worth it all

Why, then, does complexity
play such a part
For if it were easily understood
underdeveloped would be our hearts

Lord knows better than we
change builds integrity
and strength
If left up to us
we'd choose no pain
we'd go the shortest length

Learning little or nothing
gathering bits and pieces
we'd take forever learning lessons
under-qualified for God's increases

Acceptance and faith –
true keys to happiness
All things in the Master's time
Be advised His gifts are the very best

Self's Song

See the beauty that you posses
Will you caress your confidence,
finesse your acceptance
of self?
Have you embraced the supremacy of your being
blind sight could not comprehend
Did you stop and say
that God sends the perfect you,
the vital you
that can only fulfill the purpose
given you now-

And at this moment
do you embrace that you are all you need to be,
that it's not what other's see that make you who you are
but its the who that you believe that you are
that matters...
It is crucial to see that you are a beautiful being
exactly as you are
If you are not loyal to you,
then who will be?

We can only survive on other's love for so long
A song does not lack lyrics or melody
If so, it would not be a song
Love long, love hard, and love you
like you loved that person that you gave everything to,
and who scorned your soul in return...

Yearn... yes burn
then soothe
and cool take you to beautiful waters

in a pool of self acceptance
You've never had a bath like this...
Lay your head back and relax in your self confidence
that you can and will not just be
man or a woman
But that you will dent your heals
in every grain of sand possible
Residual dew will remain
from the granules poured into life
long after you're gone
Can you see why I go on and on,
encouraging you to love thine self as you are
if there is something about
you that makes you sad –
change it
because
you
are worth it
Be the best lover to you
That you've ever had

Soaking in Somber

It is the most somber
days bringing un-comparable
gifts of peace
Seek and find refuge upon a cloud
in a grey sky
Trees journeying through
Change disperse
array of color
Tepid waves of solace
is here for a time
present time basking
savoring the experience
not of what's gone by
of what can be made
of now

Soul

The sun rises in a soul
long lost soul that felt
only the coldest of winters
splinter thin icicles suspended
from chords of a vocalists
as angry verbiage and infliction
of brutality weakened an esteem

Now the sun rises in a soul
never knew the rivers
and waters were troubled
contaminated from pollution
inflicted in a tender time
a time called childhood

Who has taken the time
to listen and understand
people, yet seek to
be understood
that's just the way it is
in the "hood"

So children grow
unattended to
Bringing up themselves
attempting to create a way out

Homicide, suicide, selling
or buying drugs and guns
to use in their own neighborhood
resulting in genocide
Self hung

Somehow not all were swept
some were kept by morals
gained during that same
tender time,
keeping their heads
lifted toward the sky

Some referenced
and inquired how to aspire
despite the most
horrible circumstance

Now the sun rises in a soul

Soul's mother
danced her last dance
with a heroin shot
to her veins

What is heroic about that?

Soul's father
found dead in an ally
faced down suffocated
in his own blood

shot... because he messed
up a gangsters money
selling crack

Soul's siblings all scattered
throughout the system
yet soul kept referring back
to lessons taught earlier on
when Granny was alive

Soul chose to abide

Now the sun rises in a soul

Rise soul, rise also in the sun
reference but never look back

Sour Apples

Take a bite out of life
surprised of what's inside
bitter and sweet
warm perplexed
or cold as ice
Clichés....
plenty that make sense...
Confrontational situations
How soon do we forget

Horses brought to the well
Resistant to a drink
extend a hand
pull one up
Yet a choice is made to sink

Saving is impossible
If one refuses to be free
Easy does it...
Do not push it
simply let them be
Never made lemonade
out of lemons dealt...
Why apply heat
Knowing it easily melts
Count the blessings
let it go ... run with all
might left

Barrel half full
of sour apples
residual taste
Upon ones breathe

Red delicious apples
spoiled by a single worm
Sweet in its taste even after
it survived a storm
Search and search
until you find that
perfect, uncorrupted one
Beautiful and tasty
nourished by the sun

Splinter

Raging scream story untold
It has been lived so it must unfold
Wrinkled lines represent ones soul

Light is bright yet it's really not
Exhausted and suffocating in the dark
Threw those slabs off my back
Realized late back had cracked

Now mending...

Bending upward nice and slow
Rapidly life has began to flow
Sometimes in order to gain
One must let go

Sweet Molasses

Shedding soul
Evident change in masses
transitions from hair loss to glasses
In the cup is a thick of Molasses

Still it runneth over
Watching and feeling
The slow out pour
of destiny

sticky journey –

elevating swollen feet high
Trying not to create a mess
God's spoken word – graffiti upon ones chest
Secrets buried within one's breast

follow the words I wrote
Courageously stay

Willing to fight the foe
Is it dark or really dawn
No one has ever returned and told
Close to my break thru
Continue to carry on

The pastor preaches – you're right there
penetrating words
Child don't be overtaken by fear

A little more hope a little more time
dormant energy an undivided vine
Persevering, mind made up
Going to get to the other side-

Blindly trusting my ride...

Unsolved

Eyes only see what is physical
cannot see the unseen
Inner vision called third eye

See, It guides me, and drives me
like a sports car drives its owner
or a donor shares a piece of themselves
for the survival of another.
In this world we are not alone
We are not supposed to
underfeed the next being
instead take care of our own...
Says who?

Says the Supreme being –
Homeless men, barefoot women
that way from lack of bread
lack of another's willingness to carry
Laboring for little of nothing
Some served in the military
Then abandoned after the battle of war

A soul requires more laughing,
less grieving.
How can people breathe when
there is so much pollution
and suffocation, backbiting and hating?

I hold these acts attributable
to all men, we're all responsible
to do something
Some sit in a penthouse
eating organic grains,
sipping fine wine,
racking their brains about
stock gains

Never concerned about
those in the cellar,
slumped over with stomach pains
sleeping outdoors on
infested mattresses during
snow, sleet and salty rain.

On television the under privileged
exploited – to beg the public
for financial gains
Sure some give, those of us
That hardly have meals on our own plates

They say seventy cents a day
can buy food and school supplies
Then why are these impoverished children
still crying, still, UN-nourished

Why are their parents still dying
Why is the underlying problem still,
an unsolved equation, Why –

Millions of dollars sent to
organizations each day
Families yet, wither away
I have to say... What's going on?
First said by Marvin Gaye;

"Mother, mother there is far
too many of you crying,
brother, brother, brother,
far too many of you dying."
You know we've got to find a way;
To bring some loving here today."

Thirty-five years later, poverty
still in the same communities
Wealth remains in the same suburbs

Two eyes only see what is physical,
they cannot see the unseen.

Inner being I call my third eye
See, it guides me and drives me
like a sports car drives its owner
or a donor shares a piece of themselves
for the survival of another
Why is the underlying problem
still an unsolved equation

The Wages of Truth

You rise up in me like
a bolt of lightning
to my thorax
Born from the epitome
of my abdomen

Like rocks, molten
volcanic explosion
your disturbance brought
such corruption
then you were calm

Characteristics of a typical
storm, hmmm... normal

Do I blame? No.
Am I in pain? Yes.

Cannot pretend that
your wrath is not my own

Vacant soul echoes
lost tenant, empty home

Violation, victimization
raided the infrastructure
of our dwelling

Couldn't resist loving
the beauty of your
tornado... Sweet salt
In His image made
Are we all

I still noticed your rainbow

Now I've confessed the mess
the raging winds have caused
and am left to ponder the loss
of you entirely
and
I am
defined, just a postdiluvian

Waiting

Empty of words
parallels
Presence of thought-
Distraction of mind
Mental battle fought lesson taught
Thoughts don't just get created
They are manufactured by something
One thing or another
A present and prior discovery
Don't bother trying to
convince me...

I am in touch with my reality

Smile at me one moment
Scream at me the next instance
Cramping my existence
Natural outgoingness
Ongoing happiness.

I love you
You hide me ... deny me
Each night still sleeping beside me

Daily
Waiting for you to come
Get me from that closet
It's cold...
Dark and lonely here

Your attempt to
preserve the heat
by closing the door
isn't warm at all

I feel like the floor
you walk on

Love does make one
do crazy things, I suppose-
What are you doing today,
because me I am with you...
but alone

Doing the best you can
is what you would say
"What more do I want from you?"
Asking me so innocently....

Inside I'm crying
Blinking eyes to
prevent tears from falling
Thinking about
everything...

How long to wait?

Not just on love
but THIS LOVE
Is vanishing an option
I know I have a mind

Yet feel as though
I've misplaced my opinions
Layers of my love
un-peal like an onion
Falling harder and...
Although it gets tougher
the buffer is...
I do not shine

My soul is dull
Not do to a
lack of ambition

Rather how you drain me
Yet profess to love me
as much as I do you

I am so confused

Seems like you refuse
to just fall into me
And say...
"Forget what the world thinks."

Man, this truly stinks

When you come home
we shall address
the battles occurred
"over the wire"
you could not see

that I was just on fire for you
missing you
Wishing that
I could be with you
at this special time

Sometimes
messages are so sublime
but if you listen
they say so much

I just wanted your touch
before you left
on your trip
Maybe I would not have
vacationed in this place

Will these scabs heal?

Can you erase this?

Do you even understand?

Will you give up and walk away
because it's easy?

Will you tell me to go?

Can you handle this reality?

I guess we will soon see....

I am here still in this closet
you placed me in
where you visit me
now and again

Waiting and wanting
to just see you free and happy
like I was the first time
and each time
I see you – you see me

Stop lying to the world
and live freely
even if it is
Without me

White Collar Worker

White collar worker
So sharp and clean
Shiny black shoes
Slick and sheen

Pin-stripe suit
White shirt, blue tie
Sometimes a cap
Worn straight
never one side
Least it be a
Friday night

White collar worker

Driving your
Licorice black Benz
Rolling up to
an oval office
each morn at seven

A.M. – that is

Hand off your keys
to the maintenance man
because valet parking
don't start until ten

Nod to security
while entering
the main building

White collar worker

I have just one question
Did you kiss your wife
this morning or talk to
your children?

Window of Anticipation

Warm sighs ... waiting
Anticipating a call tonight
A voice that says, 'Come
be with me, saturate me
capture that blind side.'

Induce vision
Fine wine splashes glass
Sips, wet lips,
Crash of crystal

Curls of incense
Smoke dances above
Soft music plays
Jazz of course
Smooth silhouette
Your face
Entertaining imagery
Beauty set apart

Amazing...

How did we fall apart?

Are there any more doors
to walk through or
meadows to pick
Birds of Paradise from?

Ice to melt hot love
Apologies to accept

Warm sighs ... waiting
Anticipating a call tonight

Insensitively Intense

What I want people to know about me
Is that I am many never the same of anything
at anytime during day or night

Right now or perhaps later or if one is in between
Been told that I am "deep"...
Real straight-up and blunt
Let me not forget the most penetrating-

Intense at times

I am-

Insensitively intense...

What I want people to know
Is ... honesty is the space
from which my soul derives and...
Where it domiciles

When I give... I am giving from my core depth
Foretaste of residual affect
Sweetly honest like Honey dew is honestly sweet
Dwelling within the spirit of you to whom I speak-

I want my spirit to know you for yours to feel me.
Too many people talk just to be talking
I talk to carve a point and develop consciousness
The words that I say may create wrath within thee

Remember this is all about honesty and my sharing it with thee. What I want people to know is that I do all things with invigorating passion.

I am

Insensitively intense

So, many variations, passions... spill everywhere.

Perhaps even on you.

Splash so gently few will know. Although some just do

Folks do not realize that when they criticize, patronize, and attempt to compromise my being; they're actually validating my power. My strength is enhanced and I become more and more

Insensitively intense

I want people to know that I am about logic, living, loving, teaching and creating opportunities.

I am personable, sociable, and teachable in turn. I am a lover of soul penetrating music. My soul it must touch. I am a creator of emotions a giver of love and understanding and this few will know

And less will experience

Spirit's Quest

Soul
calling for this journey
Cannot see
Yet trust the
Dream revealed to me

Going to just spread these wings
Anticipate nothing
At the same time
Expect
ALL things while flapping

Stomp on grounds
CARVE my life print into the sand
Anointed by God's own hands
Entire body covered
In his oil
Built from the finest soil

Going to walk right into existence
Done sitting on this shelf
watching from afar

Eating observance
gained plenty
information

Deposited a lot into
hollow souls of you
Who knew?
I was developing into
A self-defined woman

Not blind of anything
Especially the
breath GOD blew into me
to accomplish so many
Great things

All in one lifetime

Here
Where I belong
My journey
Epiphany...
Finally
Living in my destiny

ABOUT THE AUTHOR

Logical Poetist (born Najai D'Raughn) has penned poems and short stories for over 30 years. She is a writer and an entrepreneur. She is the Executive Vice President of Righteous Road Enterprises, Inc., the multimedia content development company which published *Harmonic Twang*. Today she resides in Dallas, Texas where she continues to write poetry for her blog, *Najai's Cup of Cocoa*.

www.ingramcontent.com/pod-product-compliance
Lightning Source LLC
Chambersburg PA
CBHW032057150426
43194CB00006B/563